SCHIZOPHRENIA

30 Days Roadmap to Wellness

Reclaim Your Life, Renew Your Health, and Reignite Your Dreams

ELLIOT BALDWIN

CONTENTS

INTRODUCTION

CHAPTER ONE: UNDRSTANDING SCHIZOPHRENIA

1.1   What is Schizophrenia

1.2   Symptoms and Sub-types of Schizophrenia

1.3   Causes and Risk Factors of Schizophrenia

1.4   Recognizing Early Signs and Symptoms

1.5   The Prevalence and Impact of Schizophrenia

CHAPTER TWO: SEEKING PROFESSIONAL HELP

2.1   Preparing for the evaluation

2.2   Diagnosis and Acceptance of Schizophrenia

2.3   The Importance of early Diagnosis and Acceptance

2.4   Coping with Diagnosis: Understanding the emotions surrounding Diagnosis

2.5   Communicating with loved ones about Schizophrenia

2.6   Addressing stigma and overcoming negative Attitudes

CHAPTER THREE: EMBRACE POSITIVE MINDSET

3.1   The Power of Positive Thinking

3.2   Practicing Mindfulness and Medication

3.3   Building resilience and coping skills

CHAPTER FOUR: TREATMENT AND MEDICATION MANAGEMENT

4.1   The Holistic Approach to Recovery

4.2   Medication Management and Treatment Options

4.3   Psychotherapy and Cognitive-Behavioral Therapy (CBT)

4.4   Social Support and Peer Groups

4.5   Complementary and Alternative Therapies

CHAPTER FIVE: UNDERSTANDING MEDICATION MANAGEMENT

5.1   Adherence to Mediations

5.1.1   Challenges of Medication Adherence

5.1.2   Solutions to Improve Medication Adherence

5.2   Managing Side Effects Effectively

5.2.1   Communication with Healthcare Providers

5.2.2   Lifestyle Modifications and Supportive Therapies

CHAPTER SIX: LIFESTYLE CHANGES FOR WELLNESS

6.1   The Role of Nutrition in Schizophrenia

6.1.1   A balanced Diet for Mental Health

6.1.2   Food to Avoid for Healthy Life

6.1.3   Meal Planning for Optimal Nutrition

6.2   Exercise and Physical Health

6.2.1   The Benefits of Regular Physical Activity

6.2.2   Finding an Enjoyable Exercise Routines

6.2.3   Incorporating Exercise into Daily Routine

6.3   Impact of Sleep on Schizophrenia

6.3.1   Improving Sleep Hygiene and Sleep Quality

6.4   Relaxation Techniques and Stress Management

CHAPTER SIX: CONQUER SCHIZOPHRENIA: 30-DAYS ROADMAP TO WELLNESS

7.1.1   Week 1: Empowerment through Education and Support

7.1.2   Week 2: Nurturing Yourself through Treatment and Self-Care

7.1.3   Week 3: Strengthening Coping Strategies and Skills

7.1.4   Week 4: Goal Setting and Integration

7.1.5   Week 5: Integration and Lifestyle Enhancement

7.1.6   Week 6: Resilience and Continued Growth

7.2   Monitoring Progress and Celebrating Milestones

7.3   Adjusting and Maintaining Your Recovery Plan

7.3.1   Regular Communication with Healthcare Provider

7.3.2   Flexibility and Adaptation

CONCLUSION

COPYRIGHT STATEMENT

Copyright © 2023 Elliot Baldwin

INTRODUCTION

In a world where mental health issues are increasingly recognized as significant challenges, schizophrenia stands as an enigmatic and complex condition. Often shrouded in misunderstanding and stigmatization, schizophrenia can cast a shadow over the lives of those affected and their loved ones, leaving them grappling with uncertainty and fear. However, in the midst of this darkness, there is hope.

"Schizophrenia: 30 Days Roadmap to Recovery, Reclaim Your Life, Renew Your Health, and Reignite Your Dreams." This comprehensive guide is a beacon of light for individuals facing schizophrenia, their families, and friends. Drawing on the latest research, expert insights, and real-life experiences, this book embarks on a transformative journey towards recovery, resilience, and empowerment.

Within these pages, you will embark on a 30-day roadmap, carefully crafted to lead you through the multifaceted aspects of schizophrenia. We will explore the symptoms, causes, and the intricacies of this disorder, fostering a deeper understanding of its nature. With knowledge as our compass, we will navigate the challenging terrain of schizophrenia, seeking out the most effective treatments and coping strategies available.

But this roadmap is not just about symptom management; it is about reclaiming your life. Together, we will embark on a voyage of self-discovery and personal growth, uncovering the inner strength that lies within each of us. We will debunk the myths and misconceptions surrounding schizophrenia, breaking down the barriers that hinder social acceptance and support.

As we progress, we will focus on renewing your health—both mental and physical. From adopting healthy lifestyle habits to exploring innovative therapeutic approaches, we will equip you with a diverse toolkit to enhance overall well-being.

Whether you are someone directly affected by schizophrenia or a caregiver seeking guidance, "Schizophrenia: 30 Days Roadmap to Recovery, Reclaim Your Life, Renew Your Health, and

Reignite Your Dreams" promises to be your unwavering companion. It is a beacon of hope in the darkness, an anchor during stormy times, and a blueprint for transformation that proves there is a brighter, fulfilling life beyond the shadows of schizophrenia. As you embark on this empowering journey, remember that you are not alone – together, we can break down barriers, defeat stigma, and build a world where recovery and dreams are within reach for everyone.

CHAPTER ONE

UNDERSTANDING SCHIZOPHRENIA

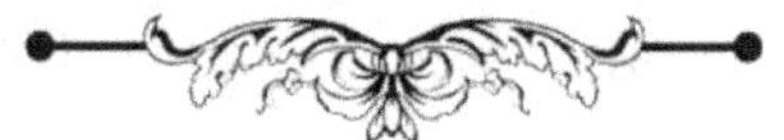

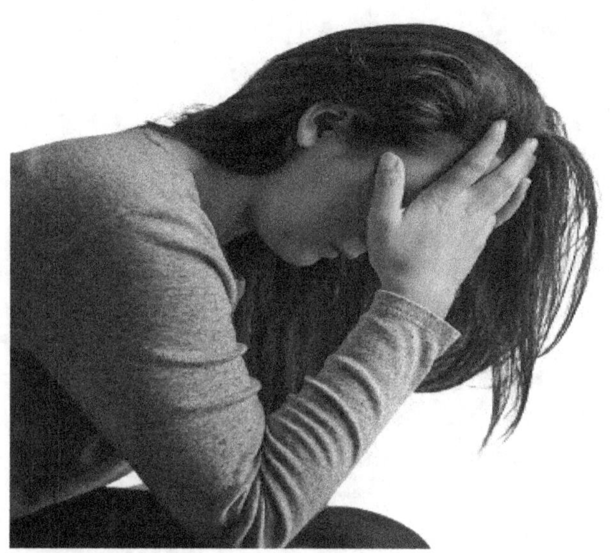

1.1 What is Schizophrenia?

Schizophrenia is a complex and chronic mental disorder that affects how a person thinks, feels, and behaves. It is characterized by a combination of psychotic symptoms, which may include hallucinations, delusions, disorganized thinking, and negative symptoms like social withdrawal and reduced emotional expression. The condition usually begins in late adolescence or early adulthood, and its causes are believed to be a combination of genetic, environmental, and neurobiological factors.

One of the key challenges in understanding schizophrenia is its heterogeneity, as symptoms and their severity can vary widely from person to person. This diversity has made it difficult to pinpoint a single cause or identify a definitive cure. However, ongoing research has provided valuable insights into the underlying mechanisms of the disorder, leading to more effective treatment approaches and improved support for affected individuals.

Genetics is known to play a significant role in schizophrenia, with family history being a risk factor. However, environmental factors such as exposure to stress, viral infections during early development, and substance abuse can also contribute to the development of the disorder. Changes in brain structure and function have been observed in individuals with schizophrenia, particularly in regions associated with cognition and emotion.

However, it's important to dispel the misconceptions and stigma surrounding schizophrenia, as this can hinder individuals from seeking help and lead to social isolation. Public awareness and understanding of the disorder can contribute to creating a more empathetic and inclusive society for those affected by schizophrenia.

1.2   Symptoms and Sub-types of Schizophrenia

Schizophrenia is a heterogeneous disorder, meaning it can manifest differently in different individuals. The symptoms of schizophrenia are generally categorized into positive, negative, and cognitive symptoms. These categories help in understanding the range of experiences and challenges faced by individuals living with the condition. Additionally, there are sub-types of schizophrenia based on the prominent symptoms and the course of the illness. Here is an overview of the symptoms and sub-types:

❖ **Positive Symptoms:**

➢ **Hallucinations:** Sensing things that are not present in reality. Auditory hallucinations (hearing voices) are the most common, but visual hallucinations can also occur.

➢ **Delusions:** Holding false beliefs that are not based on reality, often involving paranoia or grandiosity.

➢ **Thought Disorders:** Disorganized thinking, leading to difficulties in forming coherent and logical thoughts and speech.

➢ **Disorganized Behavior:** Exhibiting unpredictable or inappropriate behaviors that may not align with the situation.

❖ **Negative Symptoms**

- ➢ **Affective Flattening:** Reduced display of emotions, including facial expressions and vocal inflections.
- ➢ **Alogia:** Decreased speech output, where individuals may speak less or provide minimal responses.
- ➢ **Anhedonia:** Loss of interest or pleasure in previously enjoyable activities.
- ➢ **Avolition:** Decreased motivation to initiate and sustain purposeful activities.
- ➢ **Social Withdrawal:** Decreased desire to engage in social interactions and maintain relationships.

❖ **Cognitive Symptoms**

These affect thinking processes and can significantly impact daily functioning.

- ➢ **Impaired Memory:** Difficulty remembering and retaining information.
- ➢ **Poor Attention:** Inability to concentrate and focus on tasks.
- ➢ **Executive Dysfunction:** Challenges in planning, organizing, and making decisions.

1.2.1 Sub-Types of Schizophrenia

Schizophrenia has been traditionally classified into several sub-types, although contemporary diagnostic systems like the DSM-5 (Diagnostic and Statistical Manual of Mental Disorders) have moved away from this categorical approach in favor of a spectrum view. Nonetheless, understanding the historical sub-types can still be valuable:

- ➢ **Paranoid Schizophrenia:** Characterized by prominent delusions and hallucinations, often with themes of persecution or conspiracy.
- ➢ **Disorganized Schizophrenia:** Marked by disorganized speech and behavior, flat or inappropriate affect, and impaired daily functioning.
- ➢ **Catatonic Schizophrenia:** Characterized by severe disturbances in motor behavior, such as immobility or excessive, purposeless movement.
- ➢ **Undifferentiated Schizophrenia:** A classification used when a person does not fit neatly into any of the above sub-types but exhibits the core features of schizophrenia.

➤ **Residual Schizophrenia:** Used to describe individuals who have experienced at least one episode of schizophrenia but are currently experiencing mild or residual symptoms.

It is important to note that many individuals with schizophrenia do not fit precisely into any one sub-type, and symptoms may change over time. The current trend in diagnosis and treatment is to focus on the specific symptoms and their impact on an individual's functioning rather than rigidly adhering to sub-types. Early diagnosis, comprehensive assessment, and personalized treatment plans are crucial to effectively manage schizophrenia and support individuals in leading fulfilling lives.

1.3 Causes and Risk Factors of Schizophrenia

The causes of schizophrenia are not fully understood, but it is believed to result from a complex interplay of genetic, environmental, and neurobiological factors. While no single cause has been identified, research indicates that certain risk factors increase the likelihood of developing schizophrenia. Here are the main causes and risk factors associated with the disorder:

1) **Genetics:** Family history plays a significant role in the development of schizophrenia. Individuals with a first-degree relative (parent or sibling) who has schizophrenia have a higher risk of developing the disorder compared to the general population. However, it's important to note that having a family member with schizophrenia does not guarantee that others in the family will develop it, as genetics is just one piece of the puzzle.

2) **Neurobiological Factors:** There is evidence to suggest that abnormalities in brain structure and function contribute to the development of schizophrenia. For example, imbalances in certain neurotransmitters, such as dopamine and glutamate, may play a role in the symptoms of the disorder. Additionally, changes in brain development during early fetal life and adolescence may influence the risk of developing schizophrenia.

3) **Environmental Factors:** Various environmental factors have been linked to an increased risk of schizophrenia. These may include:

- **Prenatal and Perinatal Factors:** Infections or complications during pregnancy and birth, such as maternal infections, fetal hypoxia (oxygen deprivation), or maternal stress, may increase the risk of schizophrenia.

- **Childhood trauma:** Physical, emotional, or sexual abuse during childhood may increase the risk of developing schizophrenia later in life.

- **Urban Environment:** Growing up in urban areas has been linked to a slightly higher risk of schizophrenia, possibly due to increased stress and exposure to environmental toxins.

- **Substance Abuse:** The use of certain psychoactive substances, particularly cannabis and stimulants, during adolescence or early adulthood may increase the risk of developing schizophrenia in vulnerable individuals.

4) **Immune System Dysfunction:** Some research suggests that abnormalities in the immune system may play a role in the development of schizophrenia. Inflammation and immune-related processes have been associated with the disorder.

5) **Socioeconomic Factors:** Individuals from lower socioeconomic backgrounds may have a higher risk of developing schizophrenia, although the exact reasons for this association are not entirely clear. Stressors related to poverty, reduced access to healthcare, and social support may contribute to this link.

6) **Gender and Age:** Schizophrenia affects both men and women, but men tend to develop symptoms earlier than women. The average age of onset for men is late teens to early 20s, while for women, it is typically in the mid-20s to early 30s.

7) **Migration and Urban Living:** Some studies suggest that individuals who migrate from rural to urban areas have an increased risk of developing schizophrenia, possibly due to the stress and social isolation associated with urban living.

It's important to recognize that schizophrenia is a complex and multifaceted disorder with no single cause. Rather, it results from the interplay of various factors that differ from person to person. Identifying and understanding these causes and risk factors are essential steps in developing targeted prevention and early intervention strategies to improve outcomes for individuals at risk of developing schizophrenia.

1.4 Recognizing Early Signs and Symptoms

Recognizing early signs and symptoms of schizophrenia is crucial for early intervention and effective management of the condition. Identifying these signs can lead to timely assessment and appropriate treatment, potentially reducing the severity of symptoms and improving long-term outcomes. Here are some common early signs and symptoms to watch out for:

a) **Social Withdrawal:** Individuals in the early stages of schizophrenia may gradually withdraw from social activities and isolate themselves from family and friends. They may show reduced interest in engaging in previously enjoyed hobbies or social interactions.

b) **Changes in Emotional Expression:** Early signs may include a decline in emotional expression, with individuals showing less facial expressions, tone of voice, and gestures. They may seem emotionally flat or indifferent to situations that would usually evoke emotional responses.

c) **Decline in Academic or Occupational Performance:** A decline in academic or job performance may be evident, with individuals having difficulty concentrating, organizing tasks, and completing assignments or work-related responsibilities.

d) **Unusual Beliefs or Ideas:** Early signs of schizophrenia may include the development of unusual beliefs or ideas that seem disconnected from reality. These beliefs may involve paranoid thoughts, such as feeling persecuted or spied upon.

e) **Changes in Speech Patterns:** Individuals might display changes in their speech, such as speaking in a disorganized or incoherent manner. They may also experience difficulties in maintaining a logical flow of thoughts during conversations.

f) **Heightened Sensitivity to Stimuli:** Early symptoms may include an increased sensitivity to light, sounds, or textures, leading to heightened anxiety or discomfort in certain environments.

g) **Sleep Disturbances:** Changes in sleep patterns, such as insomnia or excessive sleep, might be early indicators of schizophrenia.

h) **Difficulty Concentrating or Remembering:** Individuals may struggle with maintaining focus, making decisions, or recalling recent events.

i) **Heightened Emotional Responses:** Early signs may involve sudden mood swings or intense emotional reactions to minor stimuli.

j) **Unusual Perceptions:** Individuals may report unusual sensory experiences, such as hearing voices, seeing things that others do not, or feeling a presence that cannot be explained.

It's essential to remember that the presence of one or a few of these signs does not necessarily indicate schizophrenia. Other medical or psychological conditions can also cause similar symptoms. However, if you or someone you know experiences these early signs and symptoms, seeking a comprehensive evaluation by a mental health professional is essential.

Early intervention and appropriate treatment can lead to improved outcomes for individuals with schizophrenia. With proper support, many individuals can learn to manage their symptoms, maintain social connections, pursue their goals, and lead fulfilling lives. If you suspect someone is experiencing early signs of schizophrenia, encourage them to seek help from a mental health professional promptly.

1.5   The Prevalence and Impact of Schizophrenia

Schizophrenia is a widespread mental health condition that affects millions of people worldwide. Its prevalence and impact on individuals, families, and communities are significant, making it one of the most challenging and disabling psychiatric disorders.

❖ Prevalence

The prevalence of schizophrenia varies across different populations and regions. According to the World Health Organization (WHO), it is estimated that approximately 20 million people worldwide have schizophrenia. The disorder typically emerges in late adolescence or early adulthood, with most cases diagnosed between the ages of 15 and 35. It affects both men and women, although men may experience symptoms earlier than women.

❖ Impact on Individuals

Schizophrenia can have a profound impact on the lives of those affected. The symptoms can be distressing and disruptive, leading to difficulties in daily functioning, social relationships, education, and employment. Individuals with schizophrenia may experience a reduced quality of life, impaired self-esteem, and a sense of alienation from society. They may face challenges in understanding and interpreting reality, making it challenging to communicate and engage with others.

❖ Impact on Families and Caregivers

Schizophrenia not only affects the individual diagnosed but also places a significant burden on their families and caregivers. Loved ones often take on the responsibility of providing care and support, which can be emotionally and physically demanding. Family members may struggle to understand the complexities of the disorder and navigate the healthcare system to access appropriate treatment and resources.

❖ Impact on Society

Schizophrenia has a considerable impact on society as well. The economic burden includes healthcare costs, loss of productivity due to disability, and potential costs related to criminal justice involvement for some individuals with untreated symptoms. Additionally, stigma and misconceptions surrounding mental illness can lead to discrimination and limited opportunities for those living with schizophrenia, further hindering their chances of successful integration into society.

CHAPTER TWO

SEEKING PROFESSIONAL HELP

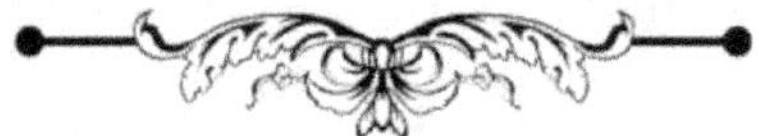

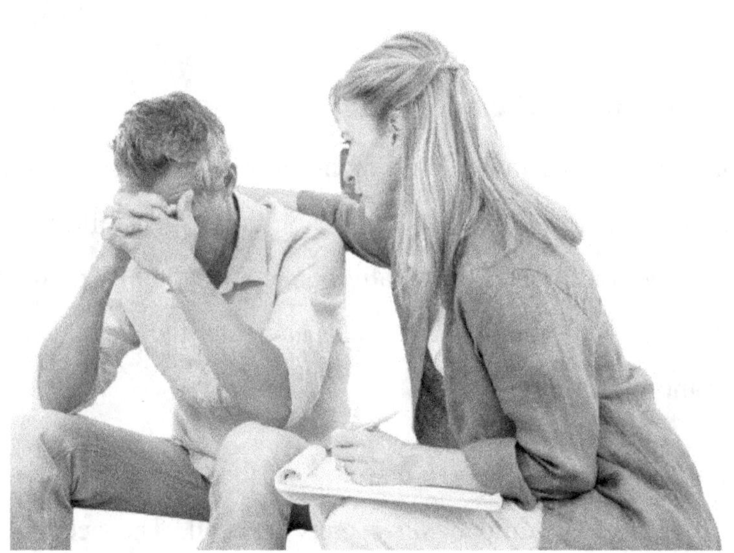

Seeking professional help is an important and proactive step for anyone experiencing mental health challenges, including schizophrenia. If you or someone you know is struggling with symptoms that may be indicative of schizophrenia or any other mental health condition, reaching out to a mental health professional is essential.

Mental health professionals, such as psychiatrists and psychologists, are trained to assess and diagnose mental health conditions accurately. Early and accurate diagnosis is crucial for developing an appropriate treatment plan and improving outcomes.

Another reason is tailored Treatment Plan, each individual's experience with schizophrenia is unique, and a one-size-fits-all approach does not apply. Mental health professionals work closely with their clients to create a personalized treatment plan that addresses their specific needs and challenges.

Remember, seeking professional help for schizophrenia is an empowering choice that can lead to improved symptom management, increased quality of life, and the pursuit of personal goals and dreams. It is an investment in your well-being and a step towards reclaiming your life, renewing your health, and reigniting your dreams.

2.1   Preparing for the evaluation

Preparing for a mental health evaluation is an important step in ensuring that you make the most out of the assessment and that the mental health professional can gain a comprehensive understanding of your needs. Here are some key tips to help you prepare for the evaluation:

a)   Gather Relevant Information

Collect any relevant information about your medical history, including previous mental health diagnoses, treatments, medications, and hospitalizations. If you have seen other mental health professionals in the past, gather their contact information and any treatment records you may have.

b)   Make a List of Symptoms and Concerns

Take some time to reflect on the symptoms you have been experiencing, any changes in your mood or behavior, and specific concerns you would like to address during the evaluation. Write them down to ensure you don't forget anything during the appointment.

c)   Be Honest and Open

During the evaluation, be honest and open about your experiences, emotions, and thoughts. The mental health professional's understanding of your situation will depend on the information you provide, so it's essential to share as much as you feel comfortable sharing.

d)   Consider Your Goals

Think about what you hope to achieve through the evaluation and subsequent treatment. Clarifying your goals can help the mental health professional tailor their approach to best meet your needs.

e)   Prepare Questions

Feel free to prepare questions you may have for the mental health professional. This can include inquiries about their treatment approach, their experience in dealing with specific conditions, and any concerns or doubts you may have about the evaluation process.

f)   Be Open to Assessment Tools

The mental health professional may use various assessment tools and questionnaires to gather more information about your condition. Be open to participating in these assessments, as they can help provide a more comprehensive evaluation.

g)   Bring a Support Person

If you feel comfortable, consider bringing a trusted support person, such as a family member or close friend, to the evaluation. Having someone familiar with your experiences can be helpful and provide additional insights.

h)   Understand the Confidentiality Policy

Familiarize yourself with the mental health professional's confidentiality policy. Understanding the limits of confidentiality can help you feel more secure in sharing personal information during the evaluation.

i)   Relax and Take Care of Yourself

Try to relax and take care of yourself before the evaluation. Engage in activities that help reduce stress and anxiety, as this can positively impact your ability to communicate during the assessment.

j)   Be Patient with Yourself

Remember that the evaluation is a starting point in the journey of understanding and addressing your mental health concerns. Be patient with yourself and the process, and trust that the mental health professional is there to support you in your healing journey.

Preparing for the evaluation allows you to be more engaged during the assessment and enables the mental health professional to develop an individualized treatment plan that meets your unique needs. Embrace the opportunity for growth and healing as you take this important step towards better mental health and well-being.

2.2   Diagnosis and Acceptance of Schizophrenia

Diagnosis and acceptance are pivotal stages in the journey of living with schizophrenia. The process involves understanding and coming to terms with the reality of the condition, which can be challenging but ultimately essential for effective management and recovery.

Receiving a diagnosis of schizophrenia can evoke a wide range of emotions, including shock, fear, confusion, and sadness. It is crucial to remember that a diagnosis is not a definition of one's worth or potential. Instead, it serves as a starting point for understanding the symptoms, accessing appropriate treatment, and finding support.

During the diagnostic process, healthcare professionals use various methods, including interviews, medical history assessments, and observation of symptoms, to establish whether schizophrenia or another mental health condition is present. Early diagnosis is valuable as it allows for timely intervention and better outcomes.

Acceptance is a gradual and transformative process that involves acknowledging and embracing the reality of living with schizophrenia. Acceptance does not mean resignation; rather, it empowers individuals to take an active role in their treatment and recovery.

Acceptance involves understanding that schizophrenia is a medical condition, not a personal failure. It involves recognizing that seeking help and support is a courageous step towards well-being. With acceptance, individuals can let go of self-blame, reduce the burden of stigma, and focus on managing symptoms and improving their overall quality of life.

2.3   The Importance of early Diagnosis and Acceptance

Acceptance is an important step towards embracing the path to recovery. By accepting the diagnosis, individuals can:

➢ **Seek Appropriate Treatment:** Acceptance enables individuals to be open to treatment options, including medication, therapy, and support services, which are vital for managing symptoms and improving quality of life.

➢ **Break Down Stigma:** Acceptance helps challenge the stigma surrounding mental health conditions, including schizophrenia. It encourages open conversations and fosters empathy and understanding within families, communities, and society as a whole.

➢ **Take Control:** Acceptance empowers individuals to take an active role in their treatment and recovery. By acknowledging the condition, individuals can better understand their needs and actively engage in self-care and coping strategies.

➢ **Build a Support Network:** Acceptance allows individuals to seek and receive support from family, friends, and mental health professionals. A strong support network can provide encouragement, understanding, and companionship on the journey to recovery.

➢ **Explore Coping Strategies:** It opens the door to exploring various coping strategies, including mindfulness, creative therapies, and self-care practices, which can enhance resilience and emotional well-being.

➢ **Moving Forward with Hope:** Diagnosis and acceptance are transformative steps that set the stage for a future filled with hope and possibility. Embracing acceptance does not mean giving up on dreams or aspirations; instead, it means integrating the condition into one's life while pursuing personal goals and passions.

Through a combination of medical treatment, psychotherapy, and support from loved ones, individuals can manage schizophrenia, reclaim their lives, and find meaning and fulfillment beyond the challenges of the condition. Each step on this journey is a testament to strength, courage, and resilience. With acceptance as a foundation, individuals can embark on a path towards recovery, wellness, and a life that is rich with possibilities.

2.4 Coping with Diagnosis: Understanding the emotions surrounding Diagnosis

The emotions surrounding a diagnosis, particularly one related to mental health conditions like schizophrenia, can be complex and overwhelming. Receiving a diagnosis can evoke a wide range of feelings, and each individual's experience is unique. Here are some common emotions that individuals may experience when facing a diagnosis of schizophrenia:

1) **Shock and Disbelief:** Upon receiving a schizophrenia diagnosis, individuals may feel shocked and have difficulty believing the news. It can be challenging to process the reality of living with a mental health condition, especially if it was unexpected.

2) **Fear and Anxiety:** Fear and anxiety are common emotional responses to a schizophrenia diagnosis. Individuals may worry about the future, how their life may change, and whether they will be able to cope with the challenges of the condition.

3) **Anger and Frustration:** Some individuals may feel angry or frustrated about the diagnosis, possibly questioning why this has happened to them. These emotions can be directed at themselves, others, or even at the circumstances surrounding the diagnosis.

4) **Grief and Loss:** A schizophrenia diagnosis can bring a sense of loss, as individuals may mourn the life, they had envisioned for themselves before the diagnosis. Grieving the loss of certain expectations and dreams is a natural part of the process.

5) **Denial and Avoidance:** In an attempt to cope with the overwhelming emotions, some individuals may experience denial or avoidance. They may avoid discussing the diagnosis or deny its implications, as a way of protecting themselves from the distressing reality.

6)   **Shame and Stigma:** Stigma surrounding mental health conditions can lead to feelings of shame or a fear of being judged by others. Individuals may worry about how their diagnosis will be perceived by friends, family, colleagues, or society as a whole.

7)   **Uncertainty and Ambiguity:** A schizophrenia diagnosis can bring a sense of uncertainty about the future. Individuals may not know what to expect, how the condition will progress, or how it will impact various aspects of their lives.

It is essential to remember that emotions surrounding a diagnosis are valid and part of a natural process of adjustment. Seeking professional support and connecting with others who have experienced similar challenges can provide a sense of belonging and reduce feelings of isolation. With time and support, individuals can navigate through these emotions, embrace acceptance, and find ways to live a fulfilling life beyond the diagnosis of schizophrenia.

2.5   Communicating with loved ones about Schizophrenia

Communicating with loved ones about schizophrenia can be a sensitive and challenging process. It's essential to approach the conversation with empathy, understanding, and patience. Here are some tips to help facilitate a constructive and supportive dialogue:

➢ **Choose the Right Time and Setting**

Select a private and comfortable environment for the conversation. Ensure there are no distractions or time constraints that could interfere with open communication.

➢ **Educate Yourself**

Before the conversation, educate yourself about schizophrenia. Understanding the condition will help you provide accurate information and dispel any misconceptions or stigma that may exist.

➢ **Be Honest and Open**

Be honest about the diagnosis and its implications, but also emphasize that schizophrenia is a treatable condition with the right support and treatment.

➢ **Use Empathetic and Non-Judgmental Language**

Use empathetic and non-judgmental language to create a safe space for open communication. Avoid blame or negative language, as it can hinder understanding and support.

➢ **Listen Actively**

Give your loved ones an opportunity to express their feelings and concerns. Listen actively and without interruption, validating their emotions and experiences.

➢ **Address Misconceptions and Stigma**

Address any misconceptions or stigma surrounding schizophrenia. Offer accurate information and emphasize that mental health conditions are no different from physical health conditions.

➢ **Offer Support and Reassurance**

Reassure your loved ones that you are there to support them and that the diagnosis does not change your relationship with them. Encourage open communication and emphasize that seeking help is a positive step towards recovery.

➢ **Set Realistic Expectations**

Set realistic expectations about the recovery process. Recovery from schizophrenia may involve ups and downs, and progress may vary. Emphasize that with appropriate treatment and support, individuals can lead fulfilling lives.

Note that each person's reaction to the news may differ, and it may take time for loved ones to process the information. Be patient, supportive, and willing to continue the conversation as needed. Communicating openly and empathetically can strengthen your relationship and foster a supportive environment for your loved ones on their journey towards recovery and well-being.

2.6 Addressing stigma and overcoming negative Attitudes

Addressing stigma and overcoming negative attitudes towards mental health conditions, including schizophrenia, requires a collective effort to promote understanding and empathy. Education is a powerful tool in dispelling myths and misconceptions surrounding mental health. By raising awareness about the realities of living with schizophrenia and sharing stories of resilience and recovery, we can challenge stereotypes and foster a more compassionate society. Encouraging open conversations about mental health and promoting a non-judgmental environment allows individuals to seek help without fear of stigma, enabling them to access the support they need for their well-being.

To overcome negative attitudes, it is crucial to engage in respectful and empathetic interactions with individuals affected by schizophrenia. Avoid using stigmatizing language or making hurtful jokes. Instead, focus on recognizing the person beyond their diagnosis and celebrating their strengths and achievements. By treating individuals with schizophrenia with dignity and respect, we can create an inclusive and supportive community that empowers everyone to lead fulfilling lives despite the challenges they may face. Together, we can break down stigma, foster acceptance, and promote a society that prioritizes mental health as an essential aspect of overall well-being.

CHAPTER THREE

EMBRACE POSITIVE MINDSET

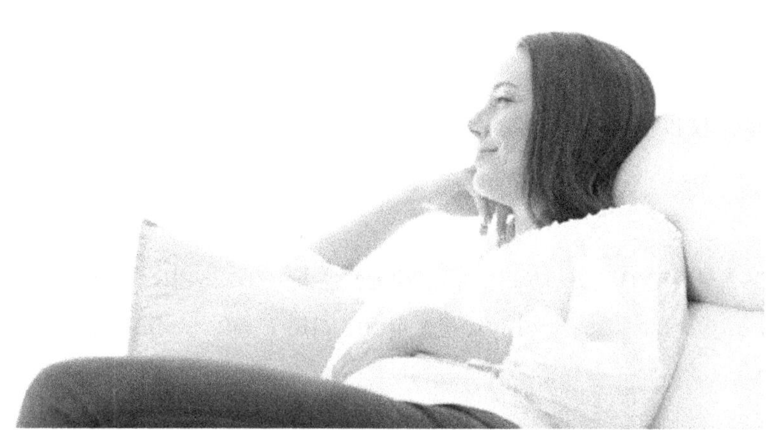

3.1   The Power of Positive Thinking

The power of positive thinking lies in its ability to shape our mindset, emotions, and actions, influencing our overall well-being and success. Positive thinking involves maintaining an optimistic outlook, even in the face of challenges and setbacks. When we embrace positivity, several benefits emerge:

a)   **Improved Mental Health:** Positive thinking can reduce feelings of stress, anxiety, and depression. It allows us to reframe negative thoughts and focus on solutions and opportunities, leading to enhanced emotional resilience.

b) **Enhanced Physical Health:** Research suggests that positive thinking is associated with improved physical health. Optimistic individuals tend to have lower stress levels, healthier coping mechanisms, and a stronger immune system.

c) **Increased Resilience:** Positive thinking helps us bounce back from adversity and persevere through tough times. It fosters a belief in our abilities and encourages us to view challenges as opportunities for growth.

d) **Better Relationships:** Positivity contributes to healthier relationships. Optimistic individuals are more approachable, empathetic, and supportive, fostering stronger connections with others.

e) **Enhanced Problem-Solving:** Positive thinking enables us to approach problems with a clear and constructive mindset. Instead of dwelling on obstacles, we focus on finding creative solutions.

f) **Heightened Productivity:** A positive outlook boosts motivation and productivity. When we believe in our abilities and remain optimistic about achieving our goals, we are more likely to take action and stay persistent.

g) **Attracting Success:** Positive thinking can attract positive outcomes. By visualizing success and maintaining a can-do attitude, we increase our chances of achieving our aspirations.

h) **Emotional Regulation:** Positive thinking helps regulate our emotions. It allows us to let go of negative thoughts and focus on gratitude and positivity, promoting emotional balance.

i) **Inspiring Others:** Optimism is contagious. When we exude positivity, we inspire and uplift those around us, creating a ripple effect of encouragement and motivation.

j) **Mindset for Growth:** A positive mindset fosters a growth-oriented perspective. Instead of fearing failure, we embrace it as an opportunity to learn and improve.

While positive thinking is powerful, it's essential to acknowledge that it is not a cure-all for life's challenges. Embracing positivity does not mean denying or suppressing negative emotions, but rather adopting a balanced approach that acknowledges both positive and negative experiences. By cultivating a positive mindset and practicing gratitude, we can navigate life's ups and downs with greater resilience, contentment, and a sense of purpose.

3.2   Practicing Mindfulness and Medication

Practicing mindfulness and meditation are powerful techniques that can enhance mental well-being and overall quality of life. Mindfulness involves being fully present in the moment, observing thoughts and emotions without judgment. Regular mindfulness practice can reduce stress, anxiety, and rumination, promoting a sense of inner peace and contentment. By cultivating mindfulness, individuals can better manage difficult emotions and cope with the challenges of daily life in a more balanced and centered way.

Medication, when prescribed and managed by healthcare professionals, can be a valuable component of mental health treatment. For conditions like schizophrenia, antipsychotic medications can help manage symptoms and improve overall functioning. Medication can reduce the intensity and frequency of hallucinations, delusions, and other psychotic symptoms, enabling individuals to engage in therapy and work towards their goals. Combining mindfulness practices with medication can create a holistic approach to mental health, addressing both biological and psychological aspects of well-being, and promoting a more comprehensive and effective path to recovery.

2.3   Building resilience and coping skills

Building resilience and coping skills are essential for navigating life's challenges, including those posed by mental health conditions like schizophrenia.

Resilience is the ability to bounce back from adversity and adapt positively to stress or difficult situations. Building resilience involves developing emotional strength, problem-solving abilities, and coping mechanisms. Individuals can cultivate resilience by fostering a positive mindset, seeking social support, and reframing negative thoughts. Embracing challenges as opportunities for growth and learning, setting realistic goals, and maintaining a sense of purpose can strengthen resilience. Resilient individuals are better equipped to face the uncertainties of life, handle setbacks, and maintain a sense of hope and optimism, even during difficult times.

Coping skills are strategies and techniques used to manage stress, emotions, and difficult situations effectively. For individuals with schizophrenia, coping skills can be particularly valuable in navigating symptoms and maintaining stability. Effective coping skills may include mindfulness practices, deep breathing exercises, engaging in hobbies or creative activities, and seeking support from mental health professionals or support groups. Coping skills empower individuals to regulate their emotions, make healthy decisions, and enhance overall well-being. By developing a diverse set of coping strategies, individuals can better manage the challenges of schizophrenia and build a foundation for a fulfilling and resilient life.

CHAPTER FOUR

TREATMENT AND MEDICATION MANAGEMENT

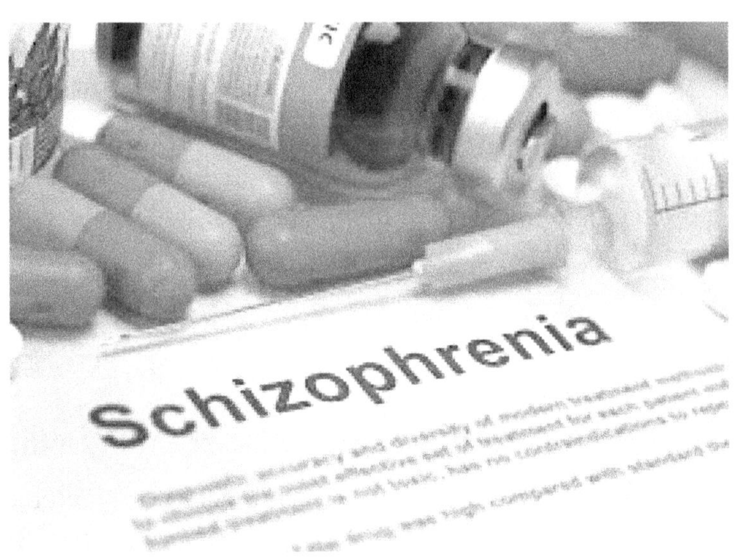

4.1   The Holistic Approach to Recovery

The holistic approach to recovery is a comprehensive and integrative method that considers the whole person – mind, body, and spirit – in the process of healing from schizophrenia. It acknowledges that mental health conditions like schizophrenia are complex and multifaceted, requiring a broad spectrum of interventions to achieve lasting recovery and well-being. The holistic approach goes beyond solely addressing the symptoms of schizophrenia; it aims to improve overall quality of life and promote self-empowerment for individuals on their journey to recovery.

> **Biological Interventions**

This aspect focuses on medical treatments and interventions, such as medication management, to address the biological aspects of schizophrenia. Antipsychotic medications can help manage symptoms and stabilize brain chemistry, reducing hallucinations, delusions, and disorganized thinking.

➤ Psychotherapy

Psychotherapy, particularly cognitive-behavioral therapy (CBT) and family therapy, is an essential component of the holistic approach. CBT helps individuals challenge negative thought patterns and develop coping strategies to manage symptoms, while family therapy enhances communication and support within the family unit.

➤ Psychosocial Interventions

This dimension emphasizes social support, skill-building, and rehabilitation. Psychosocial interventions, such as supported employment, education programs, and social skills training, help individuals regain independence and function in various aspects of life.

➤ Self-Care and Lifestyle Changes

Nurturing one's physical health through regular exercise, a balanced diet, sufficient sleep, and avoiding substance abuse can significantly contribute to overall well-being and recovery.

➤ Mindfulness and Stress Reduction

Mindfulness practices, meditation, and relaxation techniques can help individuals manage stress, anxiety, and emotional fluctuations, promoting emotional stability and resilience.

➤ Spiritual Exploration

For some individuals, spirituality or religious practices can offer a sense of purpose, comfort, and connection. Exploring and nurturing one's spiritual beliefs can be an essential part of healing.

➤ Education and Empowerment

Understanding schizophrenia and learning about one's own condition can empower individuals to actively participate in their treatment and make informed decisions about their recovery journey.

The holistic approach recognizes that each individual's experience with schizophrenia is unique, and recovery is a deeply personal process. It encourages individuals to take an active role in their treatment, advocating for their needs, and setting realistic goals. It also acknowledges the importance of family and community support in fostering a conducive environment for recovery.

By integrating various dimensions of healing, the holistic approach to recovery aims to help individuals with schizophrenia reclaim their lives, renew their health, and reignite their dreams, allowing them to thrive beyond the challenges of the disorder and find fulfillment and meaning in their lives.

4.2   Medication Management and Treatment Options

Medication management and treatment options are essential components in the comprehensive care of individuals with schizophrenia. While medication alone may not cure schizophrenia, it plays a crucial role in managing symptoms and improving overall functioning. Additionally, other treatment modalities can complement medication to enhance the individual's quality of life. Here are some key aspects of medication management and treatment options for schizophrenia:

1)   Antipsychotic Medications

Antipsychotic medications are the primary treatment for schizophrenia. They work by balancing neurotransmitters in the brain, particularly dopamine, which is thought to be involved in the development of psychotic symptoms. There are two main classes of antipsychotic medications:

a)   **First-generation (Typical) Antipsychotics:** These are older medications that have been used for decades. While effective in reducing positive symptoms, they may have more side effects, such as movement disorders.

b)   **Second-generation (Atypical) Antipsychotics:** These newer medications are generally preferred due to their lower risk of movement disorders and better efficacy in treating both positive and negative symptoms of schizophrenia.

2)   Psychotherapy

Psychotherapy, particularly cognitive-behavioral therapy (CBT), can be a valuable addition to medication management. CBT helps individuals challenge negative thought patterns, develop coping strategies, and improve problem-solving skills, enhancing their ability to manage symptoms and stressors.

3)   Long-Acting Injectables (LAIs)

LAIs represent a class of antipsychotic medications administered through injection, facilitating a continuous and gradual release of the drug over an extended duration, typically spanning from two weeks to three months. These formulations offer particular benefits for individuals facing challenges in adhering to oral medications.

4)   Coordinated Specialty Care (CSC)

Coordinated Specialty Care (CSC) is an integrated and comprehensive approach to mental health treatment that focuses on early intervention for individuals experiencing their first episode of psychosis. This specialized form of care brings together a team of mental health professionals, including psychiatrists, psychologists, social workers, and other experts, who collaborate to provide personalized and evidence-based interventions.

The primary goal of CSC is to address the unique needs of individuals in the early stages of psychosis and to facilitate their recovery and successful reintegration into their communities. The team works closely with the individual, their family, and support network to develop a tailored treatment plan that emphasizes psychotherapy, medication management, vocational and educational support, and family education and support.

5)   Assertive Community Treatment (ACT)

Assertive Community Treatment (ACT) is a highly specialized and evidence-based approach to mental health care designed to support individuals with severe and persistent mental illnesses, such as schizophrenia and bipolar disorder, in their journey towards recovery and community integration. ACT is based on the principle of providing comprehensive and intensive services directly in the community rather than in traditional clinical settings.

6) Psychosocial Interventions

Psychosocial interventions, such as individual or group therapy, social skills training, and supported employment or education programs, focus on improving social functioning, enhancing coping skills, and promoting community integration.

7) Family Therapy and Support

Involving family members in treatment can be beneficial for both the individual with schizophrenia and their loved ones. Family therapy can improve communication, reduce stress, and provide a support network for the individual's recovery.

8) Individualized Treatment Plans

Each person's response to medications is different, and finding the right medication and dosage may require a trial-and-error approach. Healthcare professionals work closely with individuals to develop personalized treatment plans that consider their specific symptoms, medical history, and individual preferences.

9) Compliance and Adherence

Consistent medication adherence is essential for the effectiveness of treatment. However, antipsychotic medications may cause side effects or individuals may feel better and stop taking their medication. It is crucial to communicate openly with healthcare providers about any concerns or challenges related to medication.

It is essential for individuals with schizophrenia to work closely with a qualified healthcare team, including psychiatrists, psychologists, social workers, and other mental health professionals, to develop a tailored treatment plan that addresses their specific needs. Open communication, ongoing evaluation of treatment effectiveness, and a supportive environment are key factors in promoting successful medication management and overall treatment outcomes for individuals with schizophrenia.

4.3 Psychotherapy and Cognitive-Behavioral Therapy (CBT)

Psychotherapy, including Cognitive-Behavioral Therapy (CBT), plays a pivotal role in the comprehensive treatment of schizophrenia. These therapeutic approaches offer valuable tools to help individuals manage symptoms, improve coping skills, and enhance their overall quality of life. Let's explore psychotherapy and CBT in detail:

4.3.1 Psychotherapy

Psychotherapy, also known as talk therapy or counseling, involves working with a trained mental health professional to address emotional and psychological challenges. It provides a safe and supportive space for individuals to explore their thoughts, feelings, and behaviors and gain insight into the factors influencing their mental health.

4.3.2 Benefits of Psychotherapy for Schizophrenia

a) **Symptom Management:** Psychotherapy can help individuals identify triggers and develop coping strategies to manage symptoms effectively. It assists in reducing the intensity and frequency of hallucinations, delusions, and disorganized thinking.

b) **Improving Emotional Regulation:** Individuals learn to identify and express their emotions, leading to better emotional regulation and a reduction in emotional distress.

c) **Enhancing Communication Skills:** Psychotherapy fosters improved communication skills, allowing individuals to express their thoughts and emotions more effectively.

d) **Strengthening Relationships:** By addressing interpersonal challenges, psychotherapy can lead to healthier and more fulfilling relationships with family, friends, and the community.

e) **Encouraging Self-Understanding:** Gaining insight into one's thoughts and behaviors empowers individuals to make positive changes and set realistic goals for their recovery.

4.3.3 Cognitive-Behavioral Therapy (CBT)

CBT is a specific type of psychotherapy that focuses on the relationship between thoughts, feelings, and behaviors. It is based on the idea that our thoughts influence our emotions and behaviors, and by identifying and challenging negative thought patterns, individuals can change their emotional responses and behaviors.

4.3.4 Key Components of CBT for Schizophrenia

a) **Thought Identification:** CBT helps individuals recognize distorted or irrational thoughts that contribute to emotional distress and maladaptive behaviors.

b) **Cognitive Restructuring:** By challenging and reframing negative thoughts, individuals can develop a more balanced and realistic perspective, reducing anxiety and stress.

c) **Skill-Building:** CBT teaches practical coping skills to manage symptoms and stressors, enhancing resilience and self-efficacy.

d) **Exposure and Response Prevention:** For individuals with specific fears or anxieties, CBT may involve gradual exposure to triggers while learning healthy ways to cope with the associated distress.

4.3.5 Benefits of CBT for Schizophrenia

➢ **Psychosis Management:** CBT can complement medication management in reducing and managing psychotic symptoms, leading to improved functioning.

➢ **Enhancing Problem-Solving Skills:** Individuals learn problem-solving techniques to address daily challenges and make better decisions.

➢ **Promoting Empowerment:** CBT empowers individuals to take an active role in their treatment and recovery, fostering a sense of control over their lives.

➢ **Long-Term Stability:** CBT equips individuals with skills that they can continue to use throughout their lives, promoting long-term stability and well-being.

It's important to note that psychotherapy and CBT should be provided by trained mental health professionals experienced in working with individuals with schizophrenia. The integration of psychotherapy with medication management and other treatment approaches can enhance overall outcomes and help individuals better manage their symptoms, improve functioning, and enhance their quality of life.

4.4 Social Support and Peer Groups

Social support and peer groups play a vital role in the recovery journey of individuals living with schizophrenia. The challenges posed by schizophrenia can be daunting, but the understanding, acceptance, and empathy found within social networks and peer groups can foster a sense of belonging and empowerment. Let's explore the significance of social support and peer groups in supporting those affected by schizophrenia:

❖ Social Support:

Social support refers to the network of family, friends, and other individuals who offer emotional, practical, and informational assistance. For individuals with schizophrenia, social support can be a lifeline, providing a safe space to express feelings, share experiences, and receive encouragement during difficult times. Key aspects of social support include:

➢ **Emotional Support:** Having someone who listens without judgment and offers empathy can provide tremendous comfort and alleviate feelings of isolation.

➢ **Practical Support:** Assistance with daily tasks, such as managing medications, attending appointments, or maintaining a routine, can be invaluable.

➢ **Informational Support:** Access to reliable information about schizophrenia, treatment options, and community resources empowers individuals to make informed decisions about their care.

❖ **Peer Support Groups**

Peer support groups consist of individuals who share similar experiences and challenges related to schizophrenia. These groups provide a unique environment where individuals can connect, relate, and learn from one another. Peer support groups offer numerous benefits, including:

1) **Understanding and Empathy:** Being in the company of others who have experienced similar struggles fosters a sense of understanding and empathy that may not be found elsewhere.

2) **Validation:** Sharing experiences and challenges with peers can validate individuals' feelings and experiences, reducing feelings of alienation and self-doubt.

3) **Learning and Coping Skills:** Peer support groups offer opportunities to learn coping strategies from those who have navigated similar obstacles, inspiring hope and resilience.

4) **Sense of Belonging:** Peer groups provide a sense of belonging and camaraderie, creating a supportive community that understands the unique challenges of living with schizophrenia.

4.5.1 Community Engagement

Community engagement involves participating in social, recreational, or vocational activities within the larger community. Engaging in meaningful activities can help individuals develop a sense of purpose and identity beyond their diagnosis. Community involvement can also reduce feelings of stigma and social isolation, promoting social reintegration.

Social support and peer groups are integral components of the recovery journey for individuals living with schizophrenia. The understanding, acceptance, and shared experiences found within these networks can be transformative, providing a sense of belonging and empowerment. Whether it's through family, friends, support groups, or community engagement, social connections offer a valuable source of strength and encouragement in the face of schizophrenia's challenges.

4.5   Complementary and Alternative Therapies

Complementary and alternative therapies (CAM) are non-conventional approaches to mental health treatment that can be used alongside traditional treatments, such as medication and psychotherapy, to support the overall well-being of individuals with schizophrenia. While these therapies may not replace mainstream treatments, they can be valuable additions to a comprehensive treatment plan, promoting holistic healing and improving quality of life. Here are some examples of complementary and alternative therapies commonly used for individuals with schizophrenia:

- **Mindfulness and Meditation**

Mindfulness practices, including meditation and deep breathing exercises, promote self-awareness and emotional regulation. Mindfulness can help individuals with schizophrenia become more present and reduce anxiety, stress, and emotional fluctuations.

- **Art Therapy**

Art therapy allows individuals to express their emotions and thoughts through creative outlets like painting, drawing, or sculpting. This form of therapy can be particularly helpful for individuals who may find it challenging to express themselves verbally.

- **Music Therapy**

Music therapy involves using music to address emotional, cognitive, and social needs. It can promote relaxation, reduce anxiety, and improve mood and communication.

- **Yoga and Movement Therapies**

Yoga and movement therapies combine physical postures, breathing exercises, and meditation to promote relaxation and reduce stress. These practices can improve physical flexibility and overall well-being.

- **Dance/Movement Therapy**

Dance/movement therapy uses dance and movement to improve emotional and physical well-being. It can help individuals with schizophrenia connect with their bodies and express emotions non-verbally.

- **Herbal Supplements and Nutritional Interventions**

Certain herbal supplements and nutritional interventions may be used in combination with traditional treatments to support mental health. However, it is essential to consult with a healthcare professional before incorporating any supplements into a treatment plan, as they may interact with prescribed medications.

- **Acupuncture**

Acupuncture involves the insertion of thin needles into specific points on the body to balance energy flow. Some individuals find acupuncture helpful in reducing stress and anxiety.

- **Animal-Assisted Therapy**

Interactions with trained therapy animals, such as dogs or horses, can provide comfort and emotional support. Animal-assisted therapy can enhance mood and reduce feelings of isolation.

It is essential for individuals considering complementary and alternative therapies to discuss these options with their healthcare providers. While many of these therapies have shown promise in supporting mental health, they may not be suitable for everyone, and individual responses can vary. Integrating these therapies into a treatment plan should be done in collaboration with healthcare professionals to ensure safety and efficacy.

CHAPTER FIVE

UNDERSTANDING MEDICATION MANAGEMENT

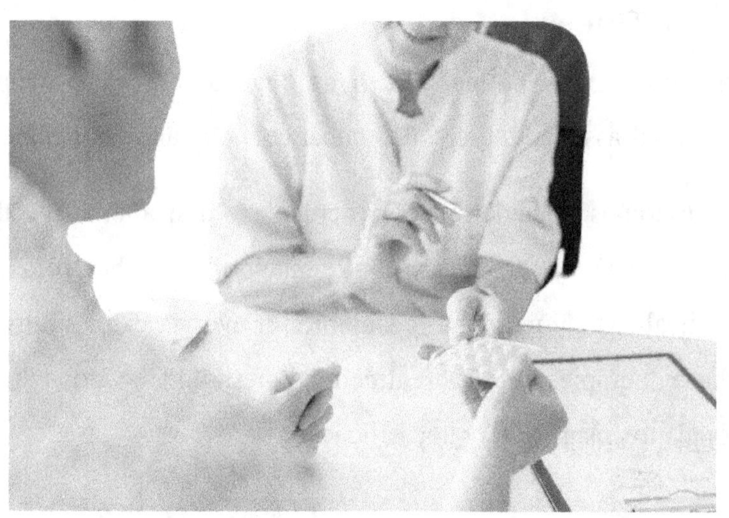

5.1   Adherence to Mediations

❖ Challenges of Medication Adherence

Adherence to medications can be challenging for individuals with schizophrenia due to various factors:

> **Side Effects:** Antipsychotic medications used to treat schizophrenia may have side effects such as weight gain, drowsiness, or movement disorders, leading some individuals to discontinue or reduce their medication.

> **Lack of Insight:** Schizophrenia can sometimes affect an individual's insight into their condition, making them unaware of the need for medication or their symptoms.

> **Stigma and Misconceptions:** Stigma surrounding mental health and medication can lead to reluctance in taking prescribed drugs due to fear of judgment or misunderstanding.

> **Complexity of Regimens:** The complexity of medication regimens can be overwhelming, particularly when multiple medications are required to manage symptoms and co-occurring conditions.

> **Cognitive Impairment:** Schizophrenia can impact cognitive function, making it challenging for individuals to remember or manage their medication schedules.

> **Substance Use:** Substance use can interfere with medication adherence and exacerbate schizophrenia symptoms.

❖ Solutions to Improve Medication Adherence

Improving medication adherence is vital for effective symptom management and overall well-being. Several strategies can address adherence challenges:

- **Education and Communication:** Providing education about schizophrenia, the importance of medication, and potential side effects can enhance understanding and cooperation. Open communication with healthcare providers helps address concerns and clarifies treatment plans.

- **Simplify Medication Regimens:** Simplifying medication regimens, such as using long-acting injectable formulations, reduces the frequency of dosing and can improve adherence.

- **Supportive Environments:** Creating supportive environments at home or in the community encourages adherence. Involving family or friends in medication management can provide reminders and encouragement.

- **Addressing Side Effects:** Healthcare providers can work with individuals to manage side effects, adjusting dosages or trying alternative medications to minimize adverse reactions.

- **Cognitive and Behavioral Strategies:** Cognitive remediation and behavioral therapies can help individuals with cognitive impairments manage their medications effectively.

- **Motivational Interviewing:** Motivational interviewing techniques can be used to explore ambivalence towards medication and enhance an individual's intrinsic motivation for adherence.

- **Integrated Treatment:** Integrating medication management with other treatments, such as psychotherapy and psychosocial interventions, provides comprehensive care and promotes overall treatment adherence.

- **Regular Follow-ups:** Regular follow-up appointments with healthcare providers help monitor medication effectiveness and adjust treatment plans as needed.

- **Address Substance Use:** Addressing substance use through counseling or substance abuse treatment can improve medication adherence and overall outcomes.

By addressing the challenges of medication adherence and implementing these solutions, individuals with schizophrenia can achieve better symptom management, improve their quality of life, and increase their chances of successful recovery.

5.2 Managing Side Effects Effectively

Managing side effects effectively is crucial for promoting medication adherence and overall well-being for individuals with schizophrenia.

❖ Communication with Healthcare Providers

Open and honest communication with healthcare providers is essential in managing medication side effects. If individuals experience any adverse reactions, they should promptly inform their doctors or psychiatrists. Healthcare providers can offer valuable insights, adjust dosages, or switch to alternative medications with fewer side effects. Regular follow-up appointments allow for close monitoring of side effects and treatment adjustments as needed, ensuring that the medication regimen is optimized for each individual's unique needs.

❖ Lifestyle Modifications and Supportive Therapies

Lifestyle modifications can play a significant role in managing medication side effects. For example, individuals experiencing weight gain may benefit from adopting a balanced diet and engaging in regular physical activity. Additionally, supportive therapies, such as cognitive remediation or counseling, can assist individuals in coping with side effects and developing strategies to mitigate their impact. Engaging in regular therapy sessions can also provide a safe space for discussing concerns related to side effects and exploring potential solutions or coping mechanisms. Through a collaborative approach that combines communication with healthcare providers, lifestyle adjustments, and supportive therapies, individuals can effectively manage medication side effects and experience better treatment outcomes.

CHAPTER SIX

LIFESTYLE CHANGES FOR WELLNESS

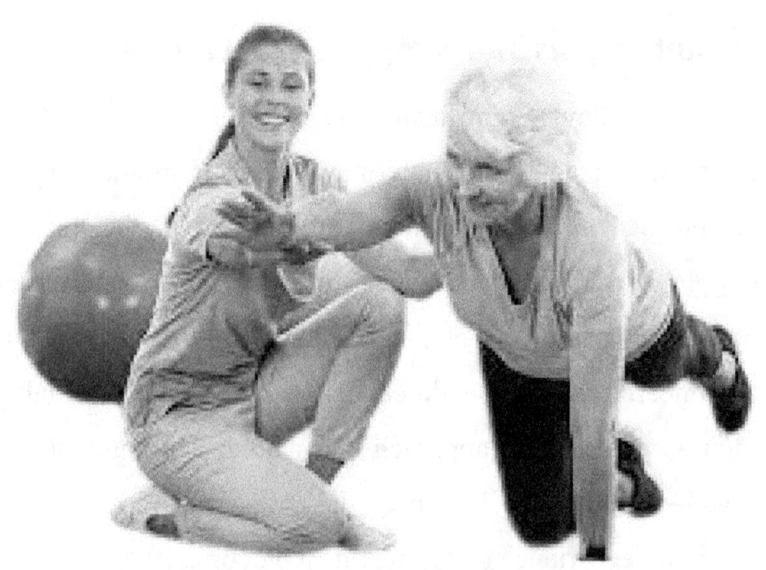

Lifestyle changes are fundamental for promoting overall wellness, especially for individuals managing schizophrenia. Incorporating healthy habits into daily life can enhance physical health, emotional well-being, and support the management of symptoms. Some key lifestyle changes include adopting a balanced and nutritious diet, engaging in regular physical activity, getting sufficient restful sleep, and reducing or avoiding substance use. Additionally, practicing stress-reduction techniques, such as mindfulness or relaxation exercises, can support emotional resilience and coping. Embracing these lifestyle changes fosters a holistic approach to wellness, complementing medical treatments and enhancing the individual's ability to navigate the challenges of schizophrenia with greater vitality and overall well-being.

6.1 The Role of Nutrition in Schizophrenia

Nutrition plays an important role in the management of schizophrenia and overall mental health. While it is not a substitute for medication or other treatments, a balanced and nutrient-rich diet can support symptom management and improve well-being. Here are some key aspects of the role of nutrition in schizophrenia:

> **Brain Health and Function**

The brain requires a wide range of nutrients to function optimally. Consuming a diet rich in essential nutrients, including vitamins, minerals, omega-3 fatty acids, and antioxidants, can support brain health and cognitive function.

> **Stability in Blood Sugar Levels**

Maintaining stable blood sugar levels is important for individuals with schizophrenia, as fluctuations in blood sugar can impact mood and energy levels. A diet that includes complex carbohydrates, proteins, and healthy fats can help stabilize blood sugar levels.

> **Reducing Inflammation**

Chronic inflammation has been linked to various mental health conditions, including schizophrenia. Antioxidant-rich foods, such as fruits, vegetables, and nuts, can help reduce inflammation and support overall health.

> **Supporting Gut Health**

Emerging research suggests a link between gut health and mental health. A diet that includes probiotic-rich foods (e.g., yogurt, kefir) and fiber can support a healthy gut microbiome, potentially positively impacting mental health.

> **Weight Management**

Some antipsychotic medications used to treat schizophrenia may lead to weight gain. A well-balanced diet can help manage weight and reduce the risk of related health issues.

> **Enhancing Medication Response**

While nutrition cannot replace medication, a well-nourished body may respond better to treatment. Certain nutrients, such as B-vitamins and omega-3 fatty acids, have been studied for their potential benefits in supporting mental health and medication response.

It's important for individuals with schizophrenia to work with healthcare professionals, including dietitians or nutritionists, to develop a personalized nutrition plan that aligns with their specific needs and medical history. Integrating nutrition as part of a comprehensive treatment approach can contribute to better symptom management, improved overall health, and a better quality of life for individuals living with schizophrenia.

6.1.1 A balanced Diet for Mental Health

A balanced diet plays a crucial role in supporting mental health, including for individuals managing schizophrenia. Here are some key components of a balanced diet that can positively impact mental well-being:

a) **Nutrient-Rich Foods:** Focus on nutrient-rich foods such as fruits, vegetables, whole grains, lean proteins, and healthy fats. These foods provide essential vitamins, minerals, and antioxidants that support brain health and cognitive function.

b) **Omega-3 Fatty Acids:** Omega-3 fatty acids, found in fatty fish (like salmon and tuna), walnuts, and flaxseeds, have been associated with improved mood and cognitive function. Including sources of omega-3s in the diet can be beneficial for mental health.

c) **Complex Carbohydrates:** Complex carbohydrates, found in whole grains, legumes, and vegetables, provide a steady source of energy and can help stabilize mood and reduce stress.

d) **Protein-Rich Foods:** Protein-rich foods like lean meats, poultry, fish, beans, and lentils support the production of neurotransmitters, such as serotonin and dopamine, which play a role in mood regulation.

e) **Hydration:** Staying well-hydrated is essential for optimal brain function. Aim to drink plenty of water throughout the day.

f) **Limit Processed Foods and Sugars:** Reduce the intake of processed foods, sugary beverages, and sweets, as they may contribute to mood swings and energy fluctuations.

g) **Moderation with Caffeine and Alcohol:** Limit the consumption of caffeine and alcohol, as excessive intake can disrupt sleep patterns and affect mood.

h) **Regular Eating Patterns:** Maintain regular eating patterns, including three meals a day and healthy snacks if needed, to keep blood sugar levels stable and support energy levels.

A balanced diet that prioritizes nutrient-dense foods can positively impact mental health, promote emotional well-being, and complement other treatments for schizophrenia.

6.1.2 Food to Avoid for Healthy Life

For a healthy life, it is important to limit or avoid certain types of foods that can have negative effects on overall well-being. Here are some examples of foods to avoid or consume in moderation:

1) **Highly Processed Foods:** Limit the intake of highly processed foods, such as fast food, sugary cereals, and packaged snacks. These foods are often high in unhealthy fats, added sugars, and sodium, and provide little nutritional value.

2) **Sugary Beverages:** Avoid sugary drinks like soda, energy drinks, and fruit juices with added sugars. These beverages can lead to weight gain, dental problems, and increased risk of chronic diseases.

3) **Trans Fats and Saturated Fats:** Limit foods high in trans fats and saturated fats, such as fried foods, pastries, and fatty cuts of meat. These fats can raise bad cholesterol levels and increase the risk of heart disease.

4) **Excessive Salt:** Reduce salt intake by avoiding salty snacks, processed meats, and excessive use of table salt. High sodium intake can contribute to hypertension and cardiovascular issues.

5) **Alcohol:** Consume alcohol in moderation or avoid it altogether. Excessive alcohol consumption can lead to various health problems, including liver disease and impaired cognitive function.

6) **Artificial Sweeteners and Additives:** Minimize the use of artificial sweeteners and food additives. While they may provide sweetness or flavor, their long-term effects on health are still a subject of research.

7) **High-Calorie, Low-Nutrient Foods:** Reduce consumption of foods that are high in calories but low in essential nutrients, such as sugary snacks and desserts.

6.1.3 Meal Planning for Optimal Nutrition

Meal planning for optimal nutrition is a strategic approach to selecting and preparing meals that prioritize health and well-being. By thoughtfully considering the nutritional content of foods, individuals can create well-balanced meals that provide essential vitamins, minerals, and nutrients necessary for overall health. Balancing food groups and portion sizes ensures a diverse and nutrient-dense diet, supporting energy levels, cognitive function, and overall vitality. By customizing meal plans to meet specific dietary goals and preferences, meal planning empowers individuals to make healthier food choices consistently, fostering a sustainable and proactive approach to maintaining optimal nutrition and enhancing overall well-being.

6.2   Exercise and Physical Health

Exercise and physical health play crucial roles in managing schizophrenia and promoting overall well-being. Engaging in regular physical activity has been shown to have significant benefits for individuals living with schizophrenia. Exercise helps to reduce symptoms such as depression, anxiety, and stress while enhancing cognitive function and memory. Moreover, it can improve sleep quality, increase energy levels, and boost self-esteem, contributing to an overall enhanced quality of life. Whether it's through structured exercise routines, outdoor activities, or simply incorporating more movement into daily life, physical activity offers a holistic approach to complement other treatments for schizophrenia. Always consult with healthcare professionals to determine suitable exercise plans based on individual needs and preferences.

6.2.1 The Benefits of Regular Physical Activity

Regular physical activity offers a wide range of benefits for individuals living with schizophrenia. Here are some of the key advantages:

- **Improved Mental Health:** Exercise has been linked to a reduction in symptoms of depression, anxiety, and stress, which are commonly experienced by individuals with schizophrenia. Engaging in physical activity stimulates the release of endorphins, the body's natural mood enhancers, promoting a sense of well-being and emotional stability.

- **Enhanced Cognitive Functioning:** Physical activity has been shown to improve cognitive functions, such as attention, memory, and problem-solving abilities. Regular exercise can help individuals with schizophrenia maintain and even enhance their cognitive skills, which can be particularly beneficial for daily functioning and overall quality of life.

- **Increased Social Interaction:** Participating in group exercises or sports activities can provide opportunities for social interaction and meaningful connections with others. Building social support networks can be vital in managing schizophrenia and reducing feelings of isolation and loneliness.

- **Better Sleep Quality:** Exercise has a positive impact on sleep patterns and helps regulate sleep-wake cycles. Improved sleep quality can contribute to better mental health and overall functioning, as sleep disturbances are common among individuals with schizophrenia.

- **Reduced Risk of Physical Health Issues:** Regular physical activity can help prevent and manage physical health issues, such as obesity, diabetes, and cardiovascular problems, which are more prevalent in people with schizophrenia due to lifestyle factors and antipsychotic medication side effects.

- **Enhanced Self-Esteem and Empowerment:** Accomplishing fitness goals and experiencing improvements in physical health can boost self-esteem and promote a sense of empowerment, leading to increased confidence in managing schizophrenia and pursuing life goals.

- **Natural Stress Reduction:** Engaging in physical activity provides a natural outlet for stress relief, helping individuals cope with the challenges associated with schizophrenia. It can serve as a healthy way to channel emotions and tension.

6.2.2 Finding an Enjoyable Exercise Routines

Finding an enjoyable exercise routine is essential to stay motivated and committed to regular physical activity. The key to discovering a routine that brings joy lies in exploring various activities and identifying those that align with individual interests and preferences. Whether it's dancing to favorite music, cycling through scenic trails, practicing yoga for relaxation, or playing a team sport, the options are diverse. Engaging in exercises that are fun and fulfilling can turn physical activity into an exciting part of the daily routine rather than a chore. Additionally, mixing up activities and trying new things can keep the experience fresh and prevent boredom. The goal is to find exercises that not only promote physical fitness but also evoke a sense of pleasure and accomplishment, making it easier to maintain consistency and derive lasting benefits from regular exercise.

6.2.3 Incorporating Exercise into Daily Routine

Incorporating exercise into the daily routine can be a beneficial and manageable approach for individuals living with schizophrenia. Start by setting realistic and achievable exercise goals that align with individual abilities and preferences. Simple activities like walking or stretching can be easily integrated into the daily schedule. Consider breaking down exercise sessions into shorter, more manageable time frames throughout the day, if needed. Engaging in physical activities that are enjoyable and can be done at home, such as dancing to music or following online workout videos, can make it easier to stay motivated. Additionally, involving a friend or family member as a workout partner can provide support and increase accountability. Gradually increasing the duration and intensity of exercises over time can help build strength and endurance while promoting a sense of accomplishment. By making exercise a regular part of the daily routine, individuals with schizophrenia can experience the many physical and mental health benefits, helping to improve overall well-being and quality of life.

6.3 Impact of Sleep on Schizophrenia

6.3.1 Understanding Sleep Disorder and Schizophrenia

Sleep disorders are common among individuals with schizophrenia and can significantly impact their overall well-being. People with schizophrenia often experience disturbances in their sleep patterns, including difficulty falling asleep, frequent awakenings during the night, and irregular sleep-wake cycles. Sleep problems can exacerbate schizophrenia symptoms, such as hallucinations and delusions, and contribute to cognitive impairments and emotional instability. Additionally, inadequate sleep can worsen daytime functioning, leading to fatigue, reduced concentration, and impaired decision-making. Understanding the complex relationship between sleep disorders and schizophrenia is crucial for providing comprehensive care and improving the overall quality of life for individuals living with this condition.

6.3.2 Improving Sleep Hygiene and Sleep Quality

> **Establish a Consistent Sleep Schedule:** Maintaining a regular sleep schedule is essential for improving sleep quality. Try to go to bed and wake up at the same time every day, even on weekends. Consistency helps regulate the body's internal clock, promoting better sleep patterns.

> **Create a Relaxing Bedtime Routine:** Develop a calming bedtime routine to signal to your body that it's time to wind down and prepare for sleep. Engage in activities that promote relaxation, such as reading a book, taking a warm bath, or practicing mindfulness or meditation.

- ➢ **Create a Comfortable Sleep Environment:** Make your bedroom conducive to sleep by keeping it dark, quiet, and at a comfortable temperature. Invest in a comfortable mattress and pillows to support restful sleep.

- ➢ **Limit Exposure to Screens Before Bed:** Exposure to screens, such as smartphones, tablets, or computers, before bedtime can disrupt sleep patterns due to the blue light they emit. Try to limit screen time at least an hour before sleep.

- ➢ **Be Mindful of Food and Drink Intake:** Avoid heavy meals, caffeine, and alcohol close to bedtime, as they can interfere with sleep. Instead, opt for a light snack if you are hungry before bedtime.

- ➢ **Get Regular Exercise:** Engaging in regular physical activity can promote better sleep quality. However, try to avoid vigorous exercise close to bedtime, as it may make it harder to fall asleep.

- ➢ **Manage Stress and Anxiety:** Practice stress-reduction techniques, such as deep breathing exercises, yoga, or journaling, to manage stress and anxiety, which can interfere with sleep.

- ➢ **Limit Naps:** While short naps can be refreshing, avoid taking long or late-afternoon naps, as they may disrupt your nighttime sleep.

By adopting these sleep hygiene practices and making them a part of your daily routine, you can improve your sleep quality and enhance your overall well-being and mental health. A restful and rejuvenating sleep is essential for maintaining physical and mental vitality and ensuring you are ready to face each day with energy and focus.

6.4   Relaxation Techniques and Stress Management

Stress and anxiety can significantly impact sleep quality. Incorporating relaxation techniques such as deep breathing, meditation, or progressive muscle relaxation can help calm the mind and promote relaxation before bedtime. Engaging in regular physical activity during the day can also improve sleep quality. Additionally, addressing sources of stress and implementing effective stress management strategies, such as therapy or mindfulness practices, can reduce sleep disturbances and enhance overall sleep health. By combining relaxation techniques and stress management, individuals can create a more peaceful and conducive sleep environment, leading to improved sleep quality and better overall well-being.

CHAPTER SEVEN

CONQUER SCHIZOPHRENIA: 30-DAYS ROADMAP TO WELLNESS

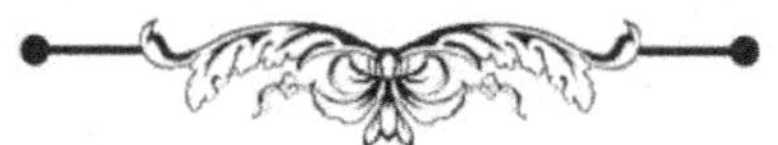

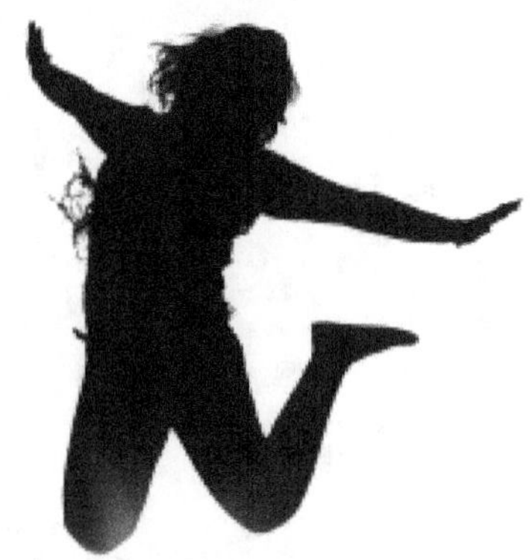

Embarking on a journey towards recovery from schizophrenia requires a well-structured and personalized plan. This 30-day roadmap is designed to support individuals on their path to freedom, offering practical steps to promote well-being and progress. Remember that recovery is a unique process, and it's essential to adapt this plan to suit your individual needs. Don't hesitate to seek guidance from mental health professionals for personalized support.

7.1.1 Week 1: Empowerment through Education and Support

➢ **Day 1: Knowledge is Power**

Take the time to research and educate yourself about schizophrenia, its symptoms, treatment options, and available resources. Understanding your condition empowers you to make informed decisions about your recovery journey.

➢ **Day 2: Seek Expert Help**

Identify and reach out to mental health professionals specializing in schizophrenia. Schedule appointments with a psychiatrist and therapist if needed. Their expertise and support are essential pillars of your recovery.

- ➢ **Day 3: Connect and Share**

Find solace in support groups, both in-person and online, where you can connect with individuals who understand your experiences. Sharing your journey and receiving encouragement can make a significant difference.

- ➢ **Day 4: Form a Support Network**

Build a reliable support network of family members, friends, or peers who can offer understanding and encouragement throughout your recovery journey.

- ➢ **Day 5: Reach Out to a Confidant**

Share your diagnosis with a close and trusted individual who can support you in your recovery efforts. Having someone who understands and stands by your side can be uplifting.

7.1.2 Week 2: Nurturing Yourself through Treatment and Self-Care

- ➢ **Day 6: Embrace Treatment**

Attend your scheduled appointments with mental health professionals and discuss your symptoms, concerns, and treatment options. Open communication with your doctor is vital for effective treatment.

- ➢ **Day 7: Medication Management**

Establish a consistent medication routine and learn about potential side effects or interactions. Transparently communicate any concerns you have with your doctor.

- ➢ **Day 8: Prioritize Self-Care**

Incorporate self-care practices into your daily routine, such as physical exercise, relaxation techniques, and a balanced diet. Caring for your overall well-being enhances your recovery process.

➢ **Day 9: Discover Mindfulness**

Explore mindfulness and meditation practices to help manage stress and foster emotional well-being.

➢ **Day 10: Restful Sleep**

Prioritize sleep hygiene by establishing a regular sleep schedule and creating a peaceful sleep environment. Adequate rest is crucial for mental health.

7.1.3 Week 3: Strengthening Coping Strategies and Skills

➢ **Day 11: Master Coping Strategies**

Learn effective coping strategies for managing schizophrenia symptoms, such as grounding techniques and cognitive behavioral therapy techniques.

➢ **Day 12: Sharpen Your Mind**

Engage in cognitive exercises or puzzles to improve focus and mental agility.

➢ **Day 13: Educate Yourself**

Participate in psycho-education programs or workshops focused on understanding and managing schizophrenia effectively.

➢ **Day 14: Skill-Building Group**

Join a skills-building group to enhance social skills, stress management, and problem-solving abilities.

➢ **Day 15: Embrace Creativity**

Engage in creative activities like painting, writing, or playing a musical instrument to express emotions and cultivate a sense of fulfillment.

7.1.4 Week 4: Goal Setting and Integration

➢ **Day 16: Reflect on Your Aspirations**

Identify your values, interests, and aspirations to set personal goals aligned with your recovery journey.

> **Day 17: Set Targets**

Establish short-term and long-term goals related to various aspects of your life, such as relationships, education, employment, or personal growth.

> **Day 18: Plan for Success**

Break down your goals into actionable steps and create a plan with specific timelines for each milestone.

> **Day 19: Take the First Step**

Begin working towards your goals, focusing on the first actionable step. Celebrate every achievement, no matter how small.

> **Day 20: Embrace Adaptation**

Continuously evaluate and adjust your goals as needed, allowing for flexibility and adaptation to changes in your circumstances.

❖ **Throughout the Journey:**

Practice self-compassion and be patient with yourself as you navigate your recovery.

Engage in regular check-ins with your support network to share progress, challenges, and victories.

Monitor and track your symptoms and overall well-being to better understand patterns and progress.

Maintain open communication with your mental health professionals, seeking guidance and adjustments to your treatment plan when necessary.

7.1.5 Week 5: Integration and Lifestyle Enhancement

> **Day 21: Assess Your Lifestyle**

Reflect on your daily routines and habits. Identify any unhealthy patterns or behaviors that may hinder your recovery and make adjustments aligned with your goals and well-being.

> **Day 22: Pursue Growth Opportunities**

Explore vocational or educational options that align with your interests and abilities. Consider part-time work, volunteering, or enrolling in courses to enhance personal growth and find purpose.

> **Day 23: Foster Social Engagement**

Engage in activities that promote social interaction and community engagement. Attend local events, join clubs or groups centered around shared interests, and practice building and maintaining relationships.

> **Day 24: Cultivate a Supportive Environment**

Create a healthy and supportive living space. Ensure your surroundings are organized, comfortable, and conducive to your well-being. Surround yourself with positive influences and eliminate stressors as much as possible.

> **Day 25: Embrace Relaxation and Joy**

Take regular breaks and practice self-care to find joy and relaxation in activities such as hobbies, spending time in nature, or pampering yourself with self-care rituals.

7.1.6 Week 6: Resilience and Continued Growth

> **Day 26: Building Resilience**

Embrace the power of resilience as you navigate setbacks and challenges. Implement strategies like positive self-talk, seeking support when needed, and reframing negative thoughts. These tools will empower you to overcome obstacles with strength and determination.

> **Day 27: Embracing Personal Growth**

Discover the path to personal growth and self-reflection. Engage in therapeutic activities like journaling, counseling, or attending personal development workshops. These practices will facilitate profound self-exploration and heightened self-awareness.

> **Day 28: Celebrate Your Progress**

Take a moment to celebrate your accomplishments and milestones achieved during your recovery journey. Recognize your resilience and express gratitude for the support and resources that have guided you on this transformative path.

> **Day 29: Inspire Others with Your Story**

Share your experiences and triumphs with trusted individuals or even a wider audience, if you feel comfortable. By opening up about your journey, you can inspire others, raise awareness, and contribute to breaking the stigma surrounding schizophrenia.

> **Day 30: Reflect and Set Intentions**

Pause and reflect on the progress you've made throughout the recovery plan. Embrace the idea that recovery is a lifelong journey, and each day offers new opportunities for personal development and well-being. Set intentions for continued growth and self-improvement.

❖ Beyond the 30 Days:

a)   Prioritize Self-Care

Stay committed to practicing self-care daily. Continue managing your medication and attending therapy sessions to support your long-term well-being. Remember, caring for yourself is essential for sustained growth.

b)   Adapt and Modify Goals

As you progress and encounter new challenges, be open to reassessing and modifying your goals. Embrace flexibility in your recovery journey to accommodate growth and changing circumstances.

c)   Stay Connected and Learn

Maintain a strong support network and engage in ongoing learning opportunities. Surround yourself with people who uplift and understand you, and seek resources that promote mental health and well-being.

d)   Advocate for Mental Health

Be an advocate for yourself and others by actively participating in mental health advocacy initiatives. Use your story and experiences to spread awareness about schizophrenia and combat stigma.

7.2 Monitoring Progress and Celebrating Milestones

As you embark on your 30-day recovery journey, it's crucial to monitor your progress and celebrate the milestones you achieve along the way. Here are some tips to help you stay on track and acknowledge your achievements:

- **Keep a Recovery Journal:** Maintain a daily journal where you can record your thoughts, emotions, and experiences throughout the process. This will help you track your progress, identify patterns, and recognize improvements over time.

- **Use Goal Tracking Tools:** Utilize digital or physical tools, such as apps or planners, to set and monitor your short-term and long-term goals. Seeing your progress visually can be motivating and give you a sense of accomplishment.

- **Regular Check-ins:** Schedule regular check-ins with yourself or with a trusted person from your support network. Use these check-ins to discuss your challenges, victories, and any adjustments needed to your recovery plan.

- **Reflect on Achievements:** Take time to reflect on the achievements you've made, even the small ones. Acknowledge your efforts and be proud of the steps you've taken towards freedom.

- **Celebrate Milestones:** Whenever you reach a significant milestone in your recovery journey, celebrate it in a way that is meaningful to you. It could be treating yourself to something you enjoy or spending time with loved ones to share your achievements.

- ➢ **Reward Yourself:** Design a system of rewards for accomplishing your goals. Give yourself something enjoyable when you complete a step in your recovery plan. These rewards can serve as positive reinforcement and keep you motivated.

- ➢ **Stay Positive and Practice Self-Compassion:** Recognize that progress may not always be linear, and there might be setbacks along the way. Be kind to yourself during challenging times and acknowledge that setbacks are a natural part of the recovery process.

- ➢ **Seek Validation from Within:** While it's essential to receive support and validation from others, learn to validate your own progress and efforts. Remind yourself that every step forward, no matter how small, is a step in the right direction.

- ➢ **Gratitude Practice:** Incorporate a gratitude practice into your daily routine. Take a moment each day to reflect on the things you are thankful for, including the progress you've made in your recovery.

- ➢ **Share and Celebrate with Your Support Network:** When you achieve a significant milestone, share it with your support network. Celebrating your successes together can strengthen the bonds and motivate you further.

Recovery is a personal journey, and progress varies for each individual. Embrace the process, stay patient with yourself, and be persistent.

7.3   Adjusting and Maintaining Your Recovery Plan

Adjusting and maintaining your recovery plan for schizophrenia is crucial to ensure continued progress and well-being.

7.3.1 Regular Communication with Healthcare Provider

Maintaining open and regular communication with your healthcare provider is vital to adjusting and fine-tuning your recovery plan. As you progress through the 30-day journey, you may encounter new challenges or experience changes in your symptoms. By discussing these developments with your mental health professionals, they can provide valuable insights and make necessary adjustments to your treatment plan. Your healthcare provider can also help you set realistic goals, offer guidance on coping strategies, and address any concerns you may have. Remember, your recovery plan should be a collaborative effort, and your healthcare provider is a critical partner in your journey to freedom.

7.3.2 Flexibility and Adaptation

As you navigate your recovery plan, it's essential to embrace flexibility and adaptability. Recovery is not a linear process, and you may encounter unexpected obstacles along the way. Be willing to adjust your goals and strategies as needed to suit your current circumstances and progress. Celebrate your successes, no matter how small, and be compassionate with yourself during setbacks. Recognize that adjusting your recovery plan does not indicate failure; it's a sign of resilience and a commitment to finding what works best for you. Stay open to learning, continue seeking support from your network, and be persistent in your efforts to overcome challenges and achieve your goals. Remember, the recovery journey is about growth and improvement, and the ability to adapt will serve you well in the long run.

CONCLUSION

As you reach the end of this 30-day recovery roadmap, it's essential to embrace your journey to wellness wholeheartedly. Remember that healing is not a linear process, and each step you've taken, no matter how small, is a testament to your strength and determination. Acknowledge the progress you've made and the milestones you've achieved, celebrating the growth and positive changes in your life.

Take time to reflect on your experiences throughout this journey. Consider the challenges you faced, the coping strategies you learned, and the support you received. These reflections will serve as valuable lessons and insights for your continued growth and well-being.

You now have the tools and knowledge to empower yourself for long-term wellness. Keep in mind that recovery is an ongoing process that requires dedication and self-compassion. Continue to prioritize self-care, stay connected with your support network, and maintain open communication with your healthcare provider. By doing so, you'll be better equipped to navigate the ups and downs of life with schizophrenia and build a resilient and fulfilling future.

As you move forward on your path to freedom, remember that your journey has the power to inspire others. By sharing your experiences and breaking the stigma surrounding schizophrenia, you can help others understand the challenges and triumphs of living with this condition. Advocate for mental health awareness and support those who may be on their own recovery journeys. Your story can be a source of hope and encouragement for many.

In closing, we want to remind you that this book is merely a guide—a stepping stone on your personal path to wellness. Your journey is unique, and we encourage you to adapt and modify the strategies outlined here to suit your individual needs. As you continue on this transformative road, know that you are not alone, and there is a community of individuals ready to support and uplift you.

Wishing you strength, resilience, and a life filled with freedom, purpose, and joy. Your journey towards wellness is a testament to the power of the human spirit.

<u>***Note to the Reader:***</u> This book is not meant to substitute for medical care, and treatment should not be based solely on its contents. Instead, treatment must be developed in a dialogue between the individual and his or her physician. This book has been written to help with that dialogue.